Healing through Milk and Yogurt

Using Dairy Products for Natural Healing

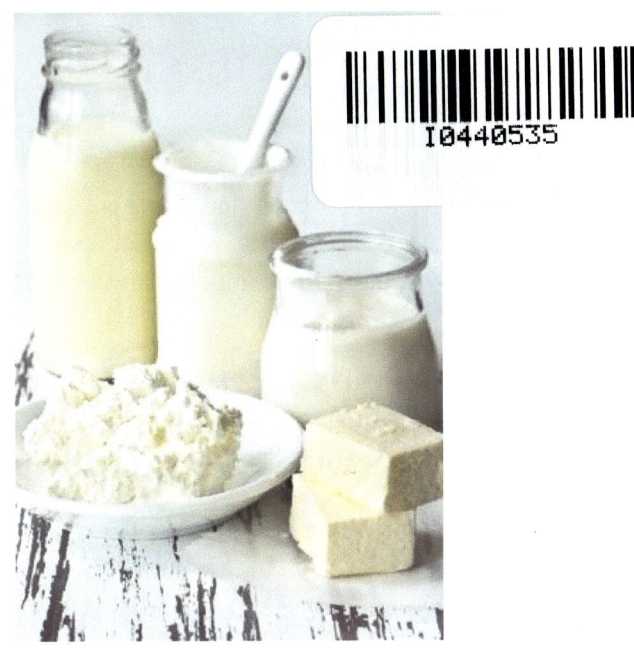

Dueep Jyot Singh

Healthy Living Series

Mendon Cottage Books

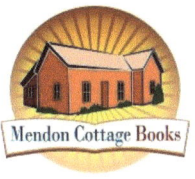

JD-Biz Publishing

Our books are available at

1. Amazon.com
2. Barnes and Noble
3. Itunes
4. Kobo
5. Smashwords
6. Google Play Books

Table of Contents

Introduction

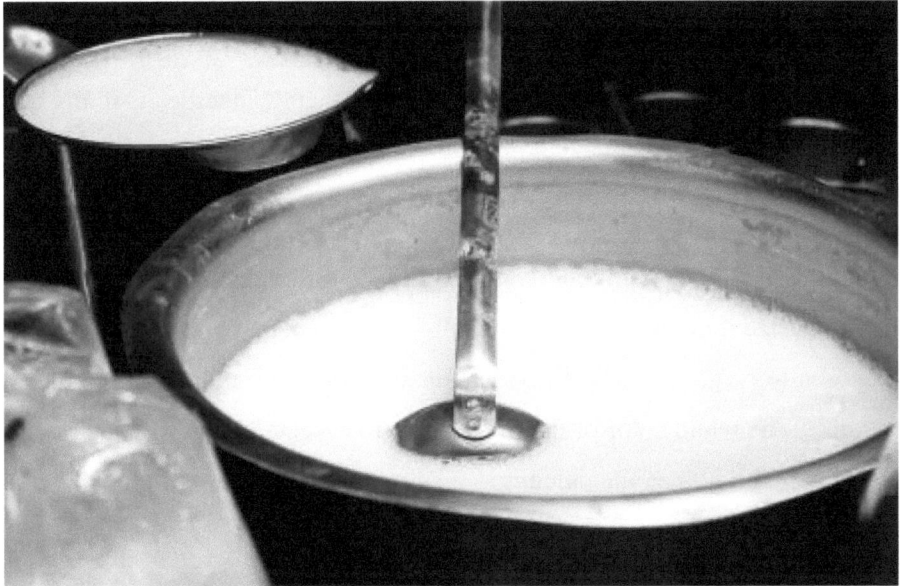

Since ancient times, mankind has considered milk from animals to be one of the most easily available and popular supplements to his diet. This milk is the main constituent of a number of other products like cheese, butter, yogurt, cottage cheese, and buttermilk. This book is going to tell you all about how you can use these products to cure a number of ailments.

In ancient times, a man's prosperity was counted by the number of livestock he had in his farm, including goats, sheep, cows, horses, and other such domesticated animals. That is why in ancient books, the milk of a cow has been described in such glowing terms –

The spinal cord of a cow has a nerve called Sunlight in it. Whenever the Sun God showers his rays on the body of a cow grazing in the fields, the rays are turned into gold when they touch the nerve called sunlight. That is the reason why the butter and the milk you get from a cow is golden in color.

Talk about imagination! But this is the reason why when the Celtic and Gaulic tribes left Britain during the Roman conquest, the women walked in front of the cows and horses in order to protect them! That means if any one tried stealing the cows away, they would have to go through the warrior women first![1]

Traditionally, milk was drank fresh without heating. It is only nowadays that we pasteurize it in order to get rid of all the germs. The yellowish color, supposed to be gold from the rays of the sun [!] is nothing but fat globules in the milk. The white color of the milk is due to casein. This is rich in nourishing and nutritional calcium.

That is the reason why growing children are given a glass full of milk morning and evening, so that they have strong bones, good teeth and a healthy constituency.

Traditionally, it is believed that the best time to drink milk is in the early morning. According to the ancients, the milk was digested as the sun went up, taking with it the benefit of the rays of the sun. That is why milk and

---

[1] And these warrior women knew how to fight, being brought up on milk, butter, and other milk products. In fact, a Roman historian of that time said, "the barbaric women of these tribes are as dangerous as their men folk. When they attack with their hands, arms and legs, shrieking, gnashing their teeth and rolling their eyes, they are a fearsome sight to strike terror in the hearts of even hardened soldiers." Incidentally, the word barbarian was used by Julius Caesar to describe these people, as equal only to sheep and baa baa- ing like them. So the term of barbarian to describe an uncultured uncivilized person, by the people of the British Isles becomes amusing.

milk products were never given to members of the family during the evening hours. There is a scientific reason behind this belief. It takes about three hours for milk to digest. That is why, if you are drinking milk at night in order to sleep more peacefully, do not go to sleep, as soon as you drink the milk.

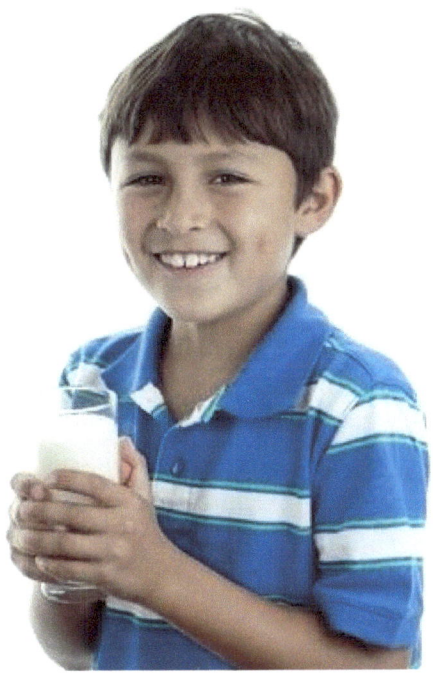

Stay awake for a while, in order to allow the milk to digest, while calming and soothing you and putting you to sleep.

Actually, the best time to drink milk at night is three hours before sleeping.

So how do you take the full benefits of milk? Fresh milk is of course supreme, but with all the infections, going around in the 21st-century world, this is not possible. That is why the milk has to be pasteurized.

There was an ancient belief, that the more you boiled the milk, the more the nutritious ingredients were lost. That is why, at that time milk was boiled only to the temperature to which you could bear drinking it down right then. This milk was sipped slowly in order to provide warmth to the body.

A friend of mine told me that her mother always whipped the milk, so that it was all foamy on top, before giving it to her children. According to her, that foamy milk was more beneficial than just ordinary milk. According to me, that foamy milk just gave me a white mustache.

Also, my friend's mother made sure that when her children were drinking a glass full of milk – foamy – in the morning, no item of their diet included anything which was sour in nature. This counteracted the effect of the milk.

That meant yogurt was never given along with a glassful of milk. Instead, it was given in the afternoon or in the evening. Yogurt is never eaten at night, though milk is drunk 3 hours before sleeping.

Most of us have the tendency of adding a spoonful of sugar to the milk, before gulping it down. This sugar milk contributes to cough and possible throat infections. Also, the calcium content in the milk gets reduced with the addition of sugar. Try drinking milk without any sugar, and appreciating its natural taste.

If you really want to add any sugar substitute or derivative, try honey, sweet fresh fruit juice, juice of raisins soaked overnight, sugarcane juice, glucose and fructose instead. Traditionally, this milk was mixed with rock candy or powdered brown sugar obtained while making molasses out of sugarcane juice. This was considered to be energy giving and strengthening.

Digesting Milk

Some people are unable to digest milk. For them, you can add a teaspoonful of honey to the milk and they are going to find it easy to digest. You can also drink orange juice along with milk or add raisins. Or you can drink a glass full of milk and eat and orange afterwards. All these are going to contribute in the easy digestion of milk without any harmful side effects and after effects.

If you think that drinking milk contributes to flatulence, try adding some pieces of raw ginger or dry ginger powder – three hefty pinches and some raisins to the milk and drink it. You are not going to suffer from any flatulence due to milk since ginger and raisins have counteracting properties to flatulence.

Also, you may try out this time-tested remedy. Take half a kilo of milk and add 250 g of grated carrots to it. Allow this to boil and then drink the milk. This is going to help in the easy digestion of the milk as well as providing you with extra iron and carotene.

Natural Remedies

Rejuvenating Recipe

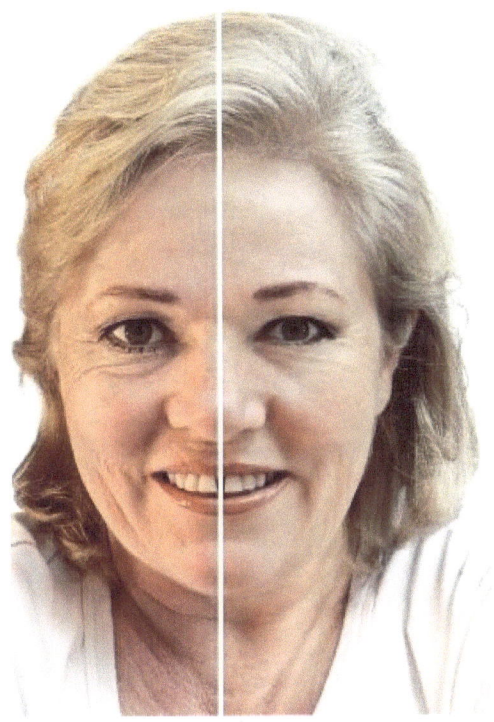

This recipe was given to me by an elder in his 80s who looks 60 and has the energy of a 40-year-old. According to him, this was a remedy, which was followed down the ages by people who definitely held onto their youth naturally with the regular intake of milk with one teaspoonful of clarified butter in it. To this they added 3 tablespoons full of honey. This was drank every night for two months every year.

And I must say, this is effective because this person look so young that no one can believe that he is hitting his 80s. His face is wrinkle free, he is strong and alert physically and mentally and he has no intention of growing old, yet!

Avoiding Milk

Many people do not know that some diseases are aggravated with drinking milk. So if you are suffering from cough, diarrhea, asthma, cramps in the stomach, stomachache, and constipation, do not drink milk until you are cured. Drinking milk aggravates cough. Instead, you should drink fresh buttermilk instead of milk, to help cure these ailments.

Increasing Weight

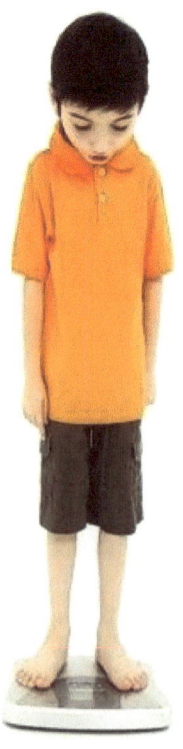

This recipe is for this little boy.

If you want to increase your weight or you think that you are not putting on the necessary weight, equal to your age, especially when you are in the growing stages, here is the traditional remedy for increasing weight.

Take a glassful of milk and add 15 raisins to it. After that, you are going to add one teaspoonful of clarified butter. Add 3 tablespoons full of honey, and drink this once a day. You are going to find yourself putting on weight, within the month.

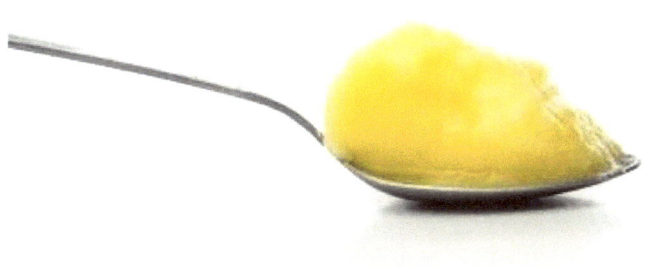

Incidentally, I was badly underweight when I was at college. I was 52 Kgs (115 pounds) at 5' 11". One of our college "workers/helpers" was a native white witch who told me that I could gain weight by eating two bananas, mashed up in yogurt, every day for three months, and 1 tablespoon full of clarified butter in one glass of milk with three spoonfuls of honey. She did not know about the raisins at that time.

Later on I found out that the raisins were added as a supplement to the milk and honey to make you put on weight even faster.

Vertigo

If you are suffering from vertigo, or a fear of heights, which makes your head spin, try adding seven raisins to 250 g of milk allowed to boil, and cool. Drink this before you go to sleep knowing that your vertigo is going to be cured naturally with milk.

Milk for Skin Problems

If you have any sort of skin ailment, you may try applying a cotton pad dipped in milk on that affected area. This is good for itches and rashes. In the same way, if you want to get rid of pimples, blemishes, and even blackheads, rub your face with hot milk, especially in the affected areas. Wash it with cold water half an hour later. This makes your skin glow.

A Scandinavian friend once told me that her mother had taught her to wash her face with salt and milk every night before sleeping to keep it fair, youthful looking, well moisturized, and without any blemishes. Thanks to her, I do that every day, and my face is totally wrinkle free even though I will never see 45 again.

Sugar remedy

When I hit my teens, my mother taught me a remedy, with which I would never ever suffer from pimples. Incidentally, I was genetically not prone to pimples, but I think that this exfoliating rub done everyday helped in keeping my teenage skin clear, glowing, and good-looking.

For this, you just need some powdered sugar. Take half a teaspoonful of this powder and make a paste with milk just enough to make it a rubbing consistency. After that, rub it gently all over your face to get rid of pimples, blemishes, spots, and other ailments.

Blemishes

If your skin is dry, moisturize it with fresh cream. If you find yourself with a wrinkled skin, moisturize it with hot milk. If you want to improve your skin tone and make it more fair, add one lemon to hot milk. This is going to curdle it. Take that curdled solid milk and apply it all over your face. This is going to cleanse it, and make you more fair.

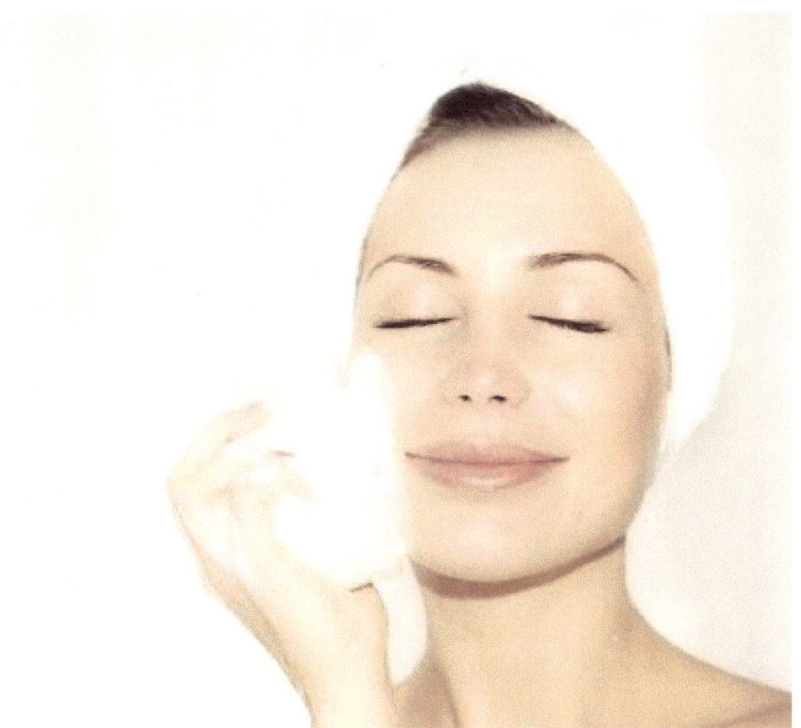

If you have blemishes on your face, rub your face for 10 minutes with this mixture. The lemon is a natural bleaching agent.

Pimples and Pimple Scars

Pimple scars are going to occur only if you have been interfering with that infected area. Unfortunately, that is something one cannot resist doing. The moment acne makes its appearance, one fiddles with it because one cannot bear the thought of that infection visible to everybody. Unfortunately, this makes the acne spread even more.

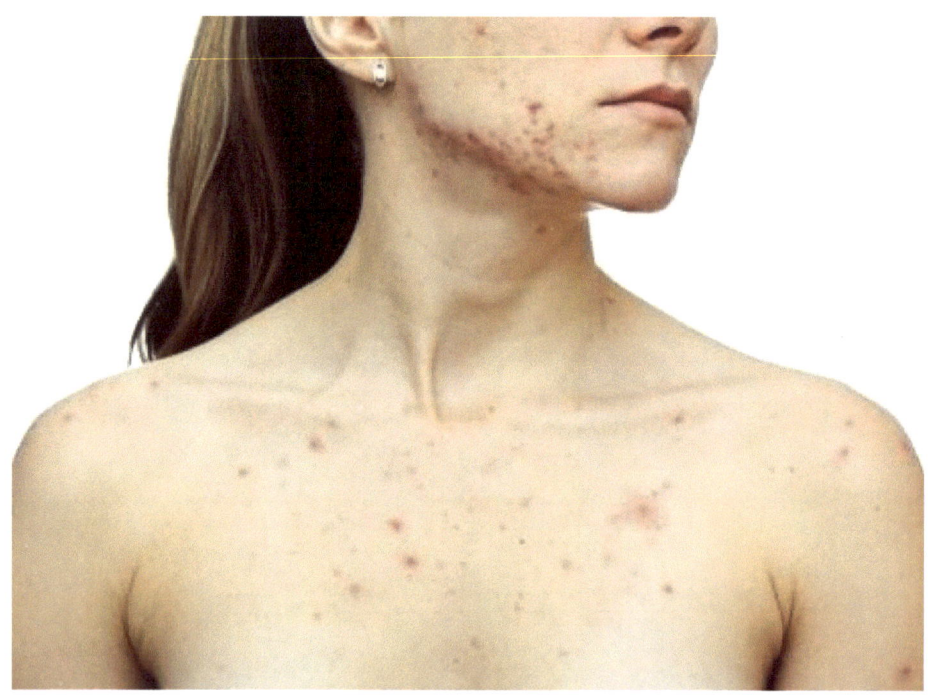

To get rid of these pimple scars, drink a mixture of water and milk in equal quantities to detoxify your body and slowly heal the skin.

If you are suffering from pimples, make up a paste of half a teaspoonful of honey, 4 teaspoons full of oatmeal, 2 teaspoons full of milk, and add one lemon to it. Now apply it all over the affected area, allowed to dry and rub off slowly with warm water. Do this regularly once a day, for a month to help heal your skin and dry up the pimples.

Natural Depilatory

When I was a baby, my grandmother made sure that she massaged my little arms and legs with a rub made up of milk and gram flour everyday, so that I never had hair growing on them, when I grew up. This is a traditional natural hair remover, for children, but as you grow old, and your skin gets tougher, you need tougher measures.

Take 5 tablespoons full of split Bengal Gram and 5 tablespoons full of Masoor dal- (lens culinaris.) This particular lentil is the staple diet of 80% of the people in the Indian subcontinent. It is also an excellent beauty enhancer.

Now take 1 tablespoon full of ground turmeric powder and just enough of milk to soak these ingredients overnight. The next morning, grind them into a paste and rub the hairy area with this cleanser. It is going to get rid of your hair, and prevent it from growing again.

If this facial hair has been caused by hormonal disturbances, especially in females, drink buttermilk made of fresh milk. This particular buttermilk is made by mixing up equal amounts of water and milk, whisked and drunk down.

Drinking this regularly for about two weeks is going to cure the hormonal imbalance and prevent the hair from growing again on the face.

Natural Cure for Baldness

Now this is one remedy, which everyone who is suffering from premature baldness is going to try out effectively. However, if your follicles have been destroyed due to overexposure to the sun and the heat, they cannot grow again. Also, if you are genetically prone to baldness, there will be a little bit of difficulty in getting your head to grow again.

This is also an excellent measure to prevent hair fall due to excess dandruff. Take six teaspoonfuls of poppy seeds. Soak them overnight in milk. The next morning, grind them up and apply them all over the affected region. Wash your hair after half an hour. This is going to promote hair growth as well as keep your hair from falling due to dandruff, and skin ailments.

Hoarse Throat and Chest Infections

This is one of my family Life savers, especially in the winter season when everybody – three generations – are prone to chest infections, due to a lowered immune system.

Take one cup of milk, 2 cups of water, one teaspoonful of ginger powder, 20 peppercorns, ground together and boil until the amount is half in quantity. Allow to cool. When it is lukewarm, add 2 tablespoons full of honey in this and drink this morning and evening, until you are cured. It is going to take about three days, if the cough is chronic. It also gets rid of the wet infection in your chest region.

 Do not ever add honey to hot milk, or heat honey, because that destroys all its beneficial qualities.

In fact, this traditional recipe was taken to the patent office in the UK, last year and was turned down with accompanying laughter and sneers because the officials there were from Asia and knew all about this remedy practiced by their ancestors. But well, somebody may try patenting this cough and cold relieving millenniums old traditional remedy, yet once again someday!

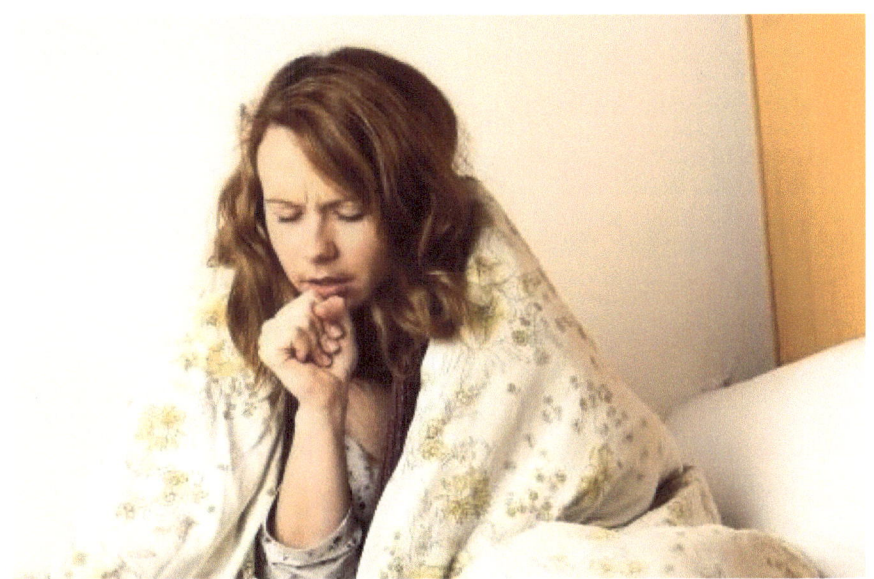

Whooping Cough

Take a mixture of one cup each of milk and water. Allow to boil until it is reduced to half. Now add half a teaspoonful of clarified butter to this mixture, and drink immediately while still hot. Do this three times a day. It takes a little while to cure the whooping cough infection, permanently and you have to do this for two weeks. You can also add some spices like powdered cardamoms and cloves to this mixture, along with honey, if you want, because they are all helpful in providing you with even more healing properties.

Acidity

If you are suffering from acidity, you need to drink cold milk, three times a day. You may also want to try out this remedy. Take one cup of hot milk and add one lemon's juice to it. The milk is going to curdle. Remove the watery portion and drink it down. The solid portion can be cooked into a tasty cottage cheese dish. The water is excellent for acidity. The cottage cheese is excellent for healing any sort of ulcers in the stomach, caused by the acid content on the inner portion of the stomach lining.

Do this every day for 15 days, and see yourself getting cured of acidity as well as stomach ulcers.

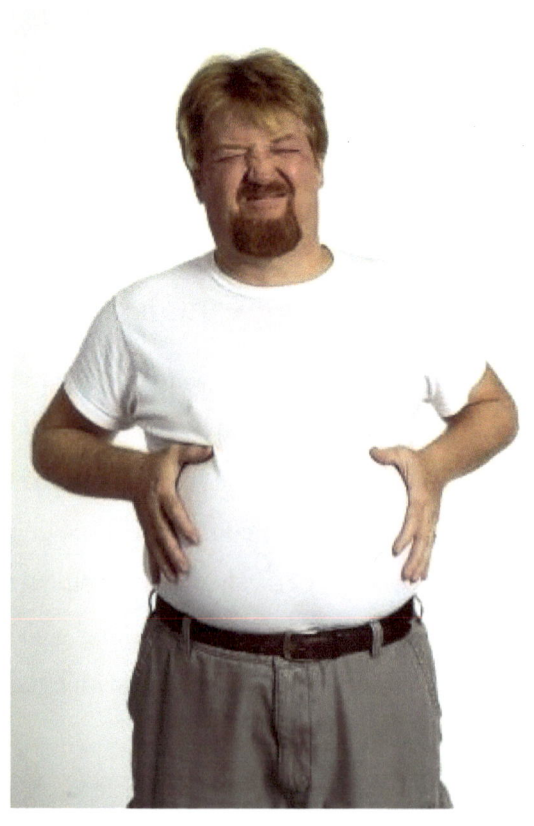

So what do you do, if your child just does not want to drink milk? It is possible, that he/she like I, has been forced to drink milk by his elders when he/she was young, with statements of, you have to drink this down, it is good for you, now be a good child. When has a child liked to drink anything which is good for him/her?

Also, when I was a baby, and would not drink milk and bring it up regularly, a doctor suggested my mother close my nose and when my mouth was opened to take some air, she had to pour down the milk down my throat. She did it once and nearly killed her baby, because the milk went the wrong way. She changed her Doctor and never forced me to drink milk again.

But those were days when doctors thought up silly stunts in order to make us drink milk. It was only when I was about seven that my father made drinking milk really interesting by making it into a competition between me and my younger four-year-old brother, about who drank milk down first, a whole glass of it, without coming up for air, and in one go itself. We did not know that this was an expert psychological way in getting us to drink milk morning and evening!

Sometimes, he alternated this particular game with another counting game in which he would count off numbers in different languages, while we drank the milk on each count. The moment he said in a number in another language, like let us say he was saying 1 – 2 – 3 – 4 in Persian and said 5 in English or in any other language, Middle Eastern, European or Asian language, we immediately caught him out with a yelled triumphant "Wrong!"

We were so triumphant about catching him, that we never knew that we had finished our glasses of milk. Enjoyable days!

So if you do not have the time to play word games with your child, because you are so busy running up to the office, and do not have the time or the energy or the inclination to make him drink his milk instead, substitute that milk with other dairy products like yogurt, buttermilk, milk- pudding, and so on. There are plenty of vitamin and mineral rich milk additives available in the market, but would you really like your children to drink bottled vitamins, when they can get the same thing from natural products like fruit and vegetables?

Also, once a child is used to milk products, he may find it not so tiring, to drink glasses of cold milk, especially when you have spiced them up with honey, powdered dry fruit, and spices.

Insomnia

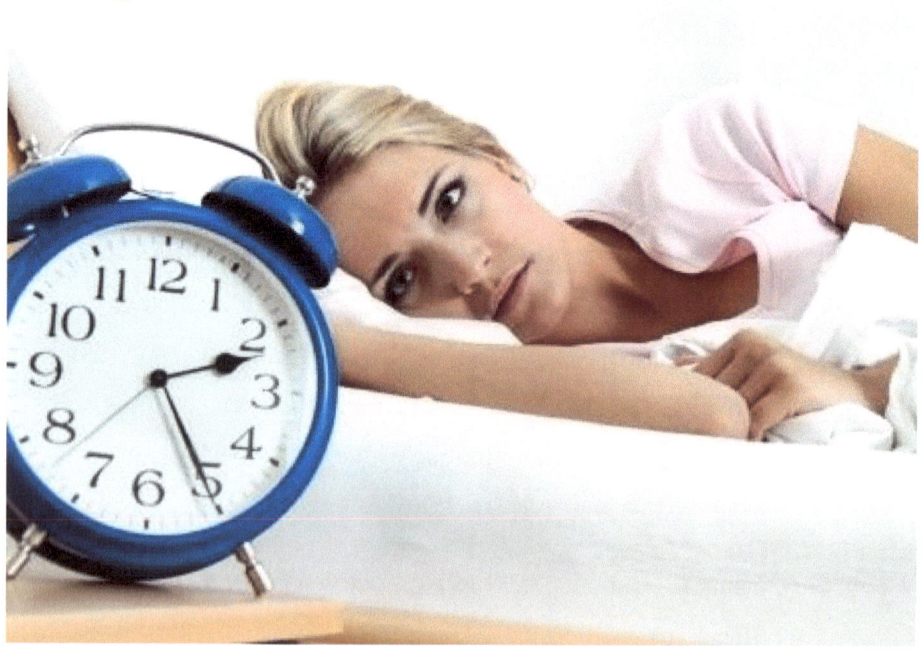

If you are suffering from insomnia, warm some milk and put a tablespoon full of honey in it. Drink it three hours before you go to sleep. You can also try eating dairy products made up of milk at dinner time in order to get a good sleep.

Almond milk

This can be drunk in summer as a cooler, and in winter, you can add a little bit of saffron to hot milk, with almonds to keep warm.

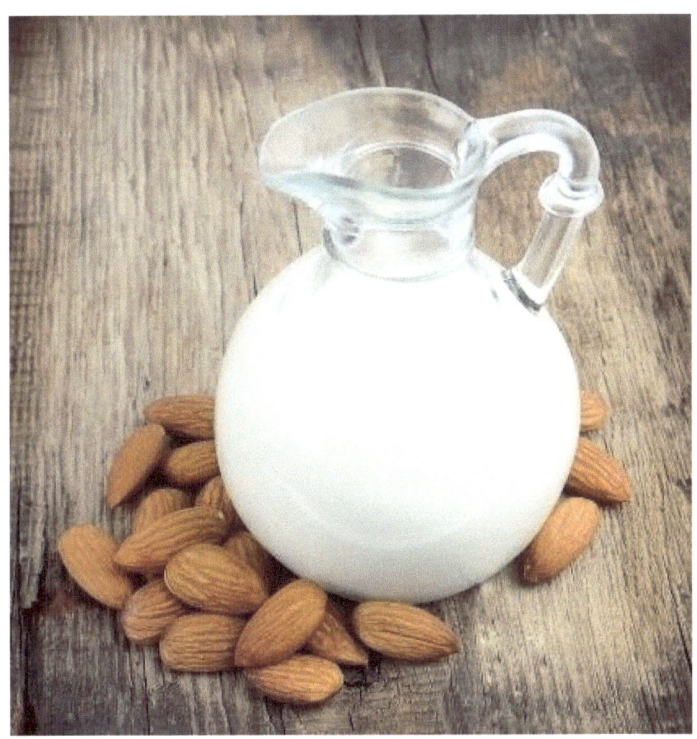

For this milk, you need 1 L of milk and hundred grams of almonds, which have been soaked overnight in water. Hundred grams of pistachios can also be added, if you are drinking it in the winter. Take enough sugar to taste, 1 tablespoon full of cream, some powdered cardamoms to spice it up, and some strands of saffron, if they are available.

Dip the saffron in 2 tablespoons full of milk, so that the color is imparted to the milk.

Put the milk on the stove to warm, and while it thickens, grind the almonds and the pistachios into a fine paste. Use the cream to make the paste. The soaked almonds are going to be easier to grind. Now add the powdered cardamoms and the sugar to this paste mixture and grind again mixing them as well. As you can.

Take off the thickened milk from of the heat, and mix this mixture in it. If you want to down it, down hot, go ahead and if you want to chill it, you can do that, also. Both ways, it is delicious to drink. Normally, in restaurants where they serve this milk, they add the saffron milk to it, to give it a saffron color and delicate taste of saffron. But that puts the price up really high!

Headaches and Migraine

Chronic migraine is a headache for people who suffer from stress and tension. Take 500 g of milk, and add 50 g of tamarind pulp to it. Tamarind is a fruit, brown when ripe, and sour in taste. Allow this to soak for one hour, and then boil the milk. The milk is going to curdle.

Ripe tamarind pulp is normally eaten, with the seeds removed.

Filter this curdled milk and take out the water. Add rock candy. According to taste to this water and drink it down. Drink this regularly once a day for a week. This gets rid of your headache.

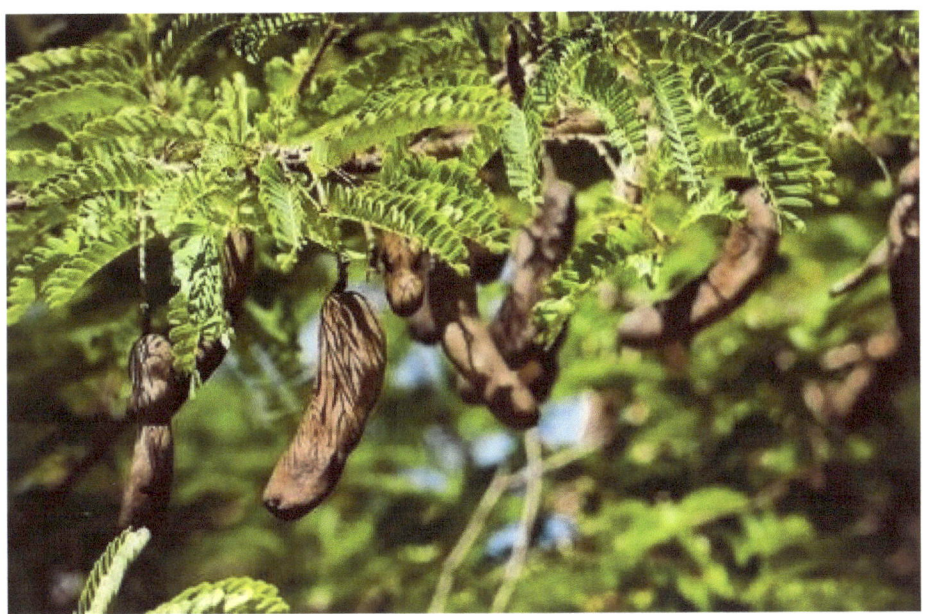

Tamarind

Along with this, here is the traditional recipe to get rid of migraines, especially for a person who has a sweet tooth.

The second one is rather amusing and very effective, because it panders to anyone with a sweet tooth.

Drink a glass full of hot milk with an accompaniment of *jalebi.*

Drink half a cup of hot *jalebi* syrup every morning, for a week. You will never suffer from a migraine ever again in your life.

For those who are not up to speed with Eastern sweetmeats, *jalebi* is a wickedly succulent and addictive dish, it is submerged into a thick sugary syrup. After five minutes , the jalebis is dripping with syrup and are taken out and drank with hot milk. This happens to be the normal breakfast appetizer of all old North Indian rustics in the winter, before they go back home to desi ghee stuffed potato pancakes.

These sweetmeats are crunchy, and filled with syrup.

How to make jalebis dripping in sugar syrup.

1 cup all purpose flour, 1 tsp besan (chickpea flour), and 2/3 cup water

For the syrup:

2 cups sugar, 2 cups water, a few threads of saffron, cardamom, and oil for frying

Combine the flours, then slowly add the water and stir. The consistency should be like pancake batter so adjust water accordingly. Stir until there are no lumps. Let this sit for 20 minutes.

For the syrup, mix the ingredients in a pot and stir over moderate heat until the sugar dissolves. Now increase the heat to high and cook uninterrupted for 5 minutes. Keep an eye on it, so that it doesn't burn.

Once the 20 minutes are over, spoon the batter into a pastry bag fitted with a plain tip 3/16" in diameter. Squeezing the batter directly into the hot oil, squeeze the batter into circular shapes, going around 4-5 times to form a sort of thin doughnut. In batches of 5-6 fry the *jalebis* for 2 minutes or until golden on both sides. As they brown transfer them to the syrup for a minute then place them on a plate. Serve warm or at room temperature.

https://www.youtube.com/watch?v=_wuJYFCN9P8

In India, sweet vendors spoon the batter into a muslin cloth with a hole through which the mixture can be squeezed. Then they use their wrist action to squeeze the spirals out into one outer circle, one inner circle and the center.

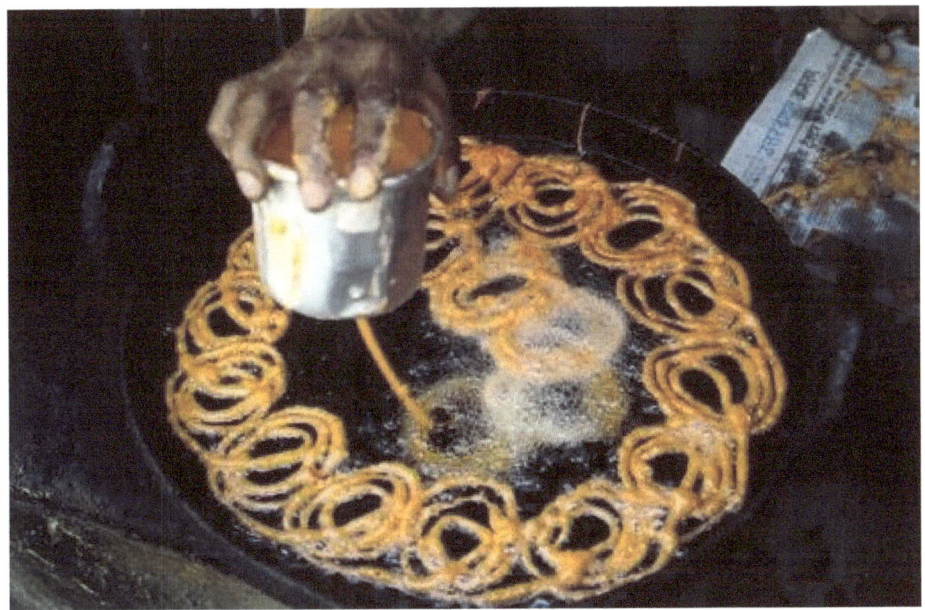

I remember walking down the streets of old Delhi one spring evening to see a very fascinated tourist couple watching jalebis being made in front of their eyes. After admiring the dexterously whirling wrist of the sweetmeat vendor, she asked him what it was called. "Jalebi , maddam ji, in English, you are calling it Round Round Stop!"

So enjoy your round round stops, and stop your migraines with its syrup or eaten for breakfast with hot milk.

It takes about one week for the migraine to disappear permanently.

Gastric and Duodenal Ulcers

A permanent cure can be achieved by putting the patient on a milk and nothing else diet. Apart from this, you can also give him pomegranate juice, and the vitamin C can be obtained from gooseberry jam. This is going to help heal him really fast.

Blocked nose

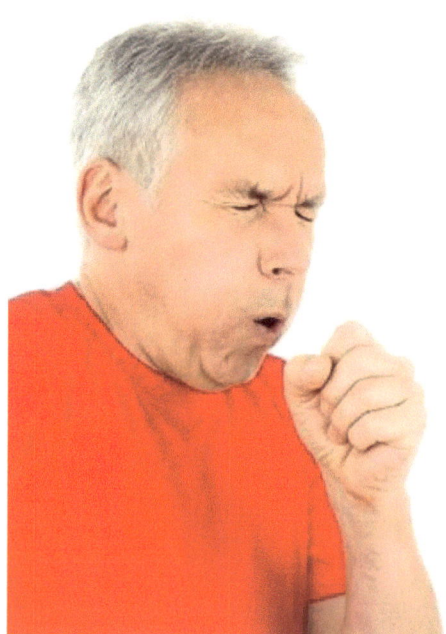

A persistent cough, especially in the winter is going to give rise to a blocked nose.

This is one remedy I tried on myself, with excellent results. I was a lifelong sufferer of chronic sinusitis and a permanently blocked nose, since childhood, ever since my nasal bones broke internally, while playing games, and blocked the nasal passage. I found this three decades later, when I went in for an x-ray! But now I have a clear nasal passage and do not have to breathe adenoid ally through my mouth.

Take one glass of milk, one glass of water, four cloves, eight small pieces of cinnamon, and boiled them all together. Allow this amount to be reduced to half when it is lukewarm, add 3 tablespoons full of honey to this and bring down. Now, cover yourself with a covering, and go off to sleep.

Do this three times a day. That means this can only be done on a holiday, when you drink milk go off to sleep. Drink milk go off to sleep. Drink milk go off to sleep. By the time you wake up the third time, definitely suffering from a sleepless night because you slept throughout the day, you are not going to have any vestiges of a blocked nose, migraine, headache, or blocked nasal passage.

Yogurt

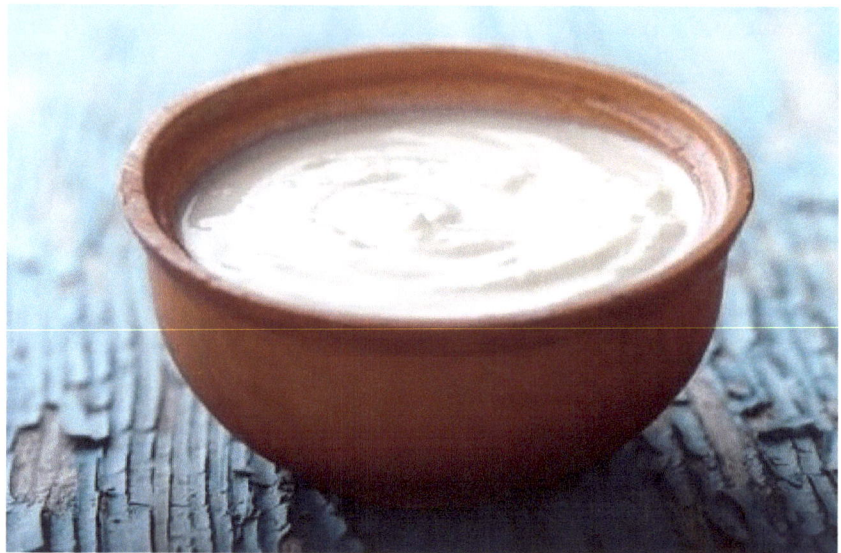

You make yogurt in the East in this traditional way. Normally, milk is boiled in India, even though you get it pasteurized. Because traditionally, Indians do not trust the pasteurizing process and would rather boil it again before use, then drink it straight from the milk bottle or from the packet.

So boil 1 L of milk. Allow to cool until it is lukewarm. You are going to see a thin layer of cream floating on top. You can keep it to add some taste to the yogurt you are making.

You need 3 tablespoons full of yogurt culture. What is yogurt culture? It is just the remainder of the yogurt, which was left behind after you finished the yogurt you made yesterday. Remember to keep at least 2 to 3 tablespoons full and do not empty out that yogurt bowl.

Dip your finger in the milk. If it is tolerably warm, in the warm weather, this is the time you put in the yogurt. Whip it briskly with a spoon, cover with a lid, and placed by one side of the stove in your warm kitchen. This is normally made overnight, so that you have perfect yogurt to eat for breakfast the next morning. The next morning, it has set, so put it in the fridge.

If you really want a traditional taste, boil this milk in a red earthernware pot, allow it to cool to lukewarm, add the culture, and leave the yogurt to set. This is considered to be one of the most delicious ways in which to eat milk products and meat products in India, and also in other countries in the East – cooking in earthenware pots. This yogurt is going to have the taste of mother Earth, in a sweetened form. I still cannot understand how that yogurt got sweet. I never added any sugar to it. It is also going to have a distinctly delicious wet earthenware aroma.

Also, I found a friend setting yogurt in cold weather, – freezing Missouri weather – by warming up her oven to 125°C for five minutes. Then she put in the yogurt container in the oven and left it overnight. Good idea!

Have you just spooned off a chunk of yogurt, only to find the rest of it turning watery? This is going to happen when you cut into the yogurt, just like you were cutting into a pie or into the cake. The best way to prevent your beautifully set yogurt from getting watery is to spoon off the yogurt, layer by layer. That means that you are spooning off the set yogurt instead of breaking it. That breaking process means you are mixing it with its watery composition and component.

According to research, yogurt has 18% more calcium than what is found in ordinary milk. For all those people who cannot digest milk, yogurt is the most nutritious diet food.

People suffering from asthma, respiratory problems, cough, and fever should not be given yogurt to eat. It should also not be eaten at night.

Lethargy

If you are suffering from lethargy, make buttermilk out of yogurt, and drink it every day. This gives you energy and also keeps your digestive system.

Constipation

If you are suffering from constipation, roast some ground cumin seeds, salt, and black pepper together. Now sprinkle this powdered powder with a peppers cellar all over your bowl of yogurt. Eat this everyday with your lunch, and you are never going to suffer from digestive problems or constipation, ever again. If you are suffering from acidity, do not allow the yogurt to get sour before you eat it. It should be eaten fresh and "sweet", before it is allowed to get sour, which is what is going to happen when yogurt gets stale.

People suffering from migraines can eat a mixture of yogurt, rice, and rock candy first thing in the morning. Eat this for at least six days.

I remember going to a friend's house, to pick her up before our final exams in high school. Her mother immediately fed the both of us with a bowlful of yogurt with honey mixed in it, because she said we needed to keep our cool. We aced our examinations. Naturally, we had studied really hard, but yogurt and honey gave us plenty of energy during the three hour long grueling session which would either make or break us, those results being counted upper most towards our college admissions.

The Best Way to Eat Yogurt

This is a natural way in which yogurt should be eaten take fresh yogurt and add honey or molasses to it. Add a little water to this mixture. This was actually eaten at Dawn by the ancients during the first meal of the day, at Dawn break. The water was added to it to give it more power. The honey was an energy giving supplement.

If your yogurt gets sour, just tie it in a muslin cloth, and hang it over a utensil. The water is going to drip out of it and the sourness is going to be removed.

Yogurt for Hair Care

Hair fall

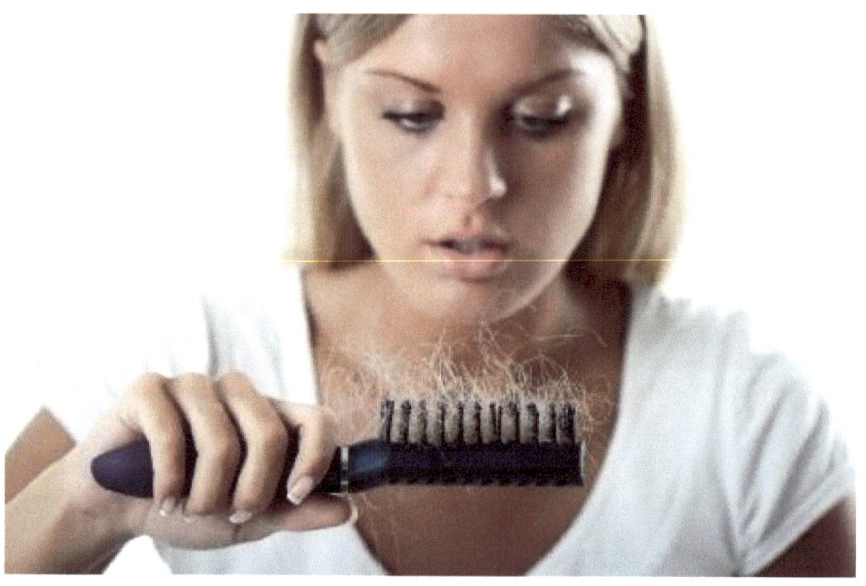

Remember that you lose about a hundred hairs from your head, daily. Naturally, that is because they have to make room for a fresher head of hair. Do not get stressed and tense like the Empress of Austria, Sisi , who used to get her hair brushed three times a day, and yell at her ladies in waiting, because a hair had fallen out. In fact, she was so neurotic that she made them stick the hair on to her scalp so that she could persuade herself that the hair had not fallen out.

Do not get stressed if you find your hair falling out. They may fall out due to tension, and you get stressed because they are falling out due to stress and tension, and this is going to be a vicious circle. Instead, increase your iron content, vitamin B, and iodine quotient in your meals. Wash your hair with yogurt. This keeps your hair healthy.

This hair washing and shampooing is done by applying yogurt to the roots of your hair. This nourishes your hair. Let us say for half an hour, and then wash your hair with water. Do not shampoo it with any other soap or shampoo. Your hair is now clean, and well nourished.

If you want to keep your hair dark – this is not for blondes and redheads – you are going to put one lemon in half a cup of yogurt. Rub this mixture all over the roots of your hair, and over your hair. This should be allowed to stay on for 20 minutes before you shampoo them. This is a natural hair darkener and hair moisturizer. You will not need to condition your hair afterwards.

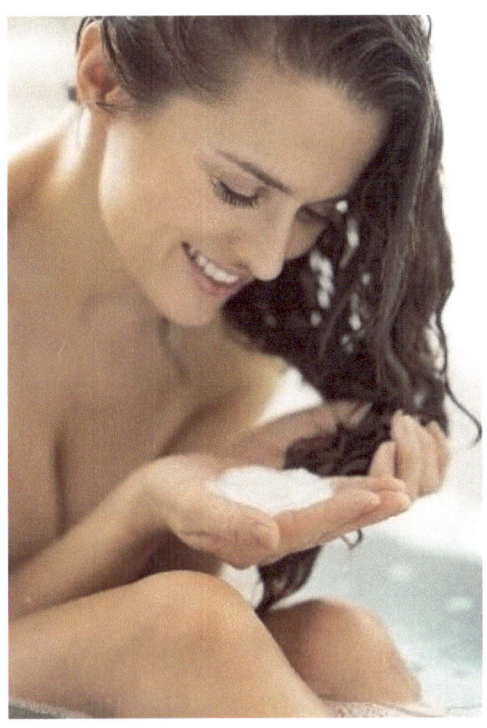

You can also keep your hair dark by putting 10 ground peppercorns in one cup of yogurt. This is excellent for cleaning your hair and keeping them shiny, dark, and healthy. This also prevents hair fall. You need to do this shampoo once a week.

Dandruff

Dandruff is the superficial dead skin of your scalp, which sloughs off every seven days. It is rather itchy, and that is why people keep looking for chemical shampoo in order to get rid of that dandruff.

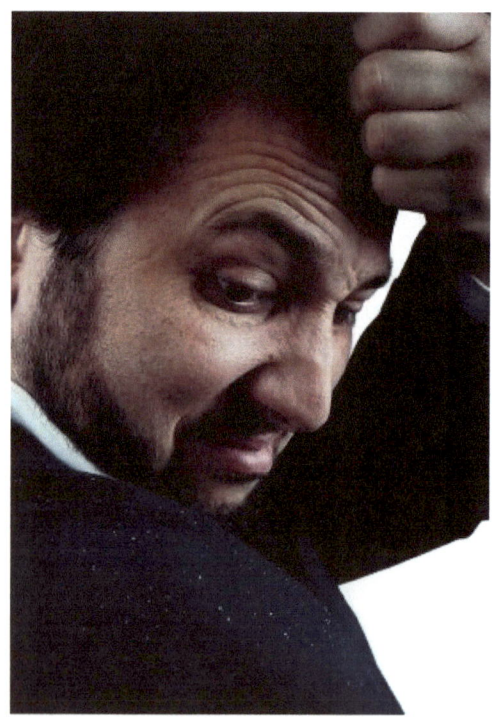

This dandruff can also affect the whole of your body and you are going to find yourself itching and scratching your arms and legs. After all, it is dry skin. To get rid of this, you are going to add 3 tablespoons full of molasses to 1 cup of yogurt. This makes a powerful antidote to dandruff.

Apply it all over the affected areas on your scalp. Wash your hair after 30 minutes. This is going to get rid of all the dandruff.

Instead of molasses, which may not be readily available, you can also get a cure by adding 2 tablespoons full of salt to 1 cup of yogurt. Rub your hair and scalp with this shampoo. The salt is going to get rid of all the dandruff.

Yogurt for Beauty

Yogurt has long been known to be an excellent beauty agent, because after all, it has milk in it, especially fermented milk, and it has also skin whitening properties.

Skin Cleansing

Do this skin cleansing, every day before you go to sleep, by mixing one teaspoonful of lemon juice in one spoonful of yogurt. Dip a cotton swab in it, and apply it all over your skin get rid of the dirt and the grime by rubbing this swab all over your face, neck, and even on your hands in circular motions. This also keeps your skin smooth, dirt free, and well moisturized.

You can also put a teaspoonful of salt, and yogurt, and rub it all over your face, before going to sleep as a cleansing lotion. This gets rid of all the dirt and dead cells.

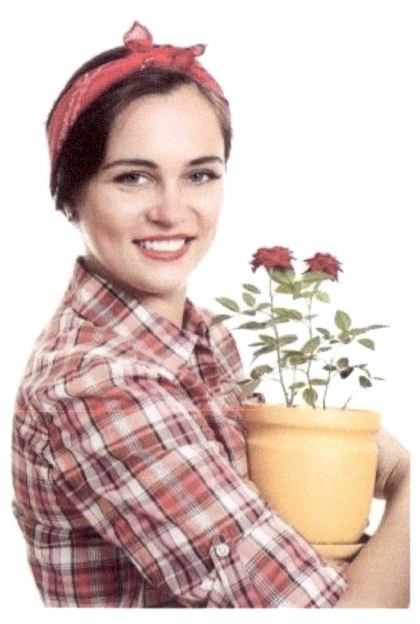

Blemishes and Pimples

If you find yourself suffering from skin blemishes, especially due to sunburn or sun damage, apply yogurt on your body like a scrub. Get rid of all the dirt, and have a shower after five minutes. Do not use any other soap or bubble bath.

This gets rid of pimples as well as blemishes, when used regularly.

Traditional Clarified Butter – Desi Ghee

Desi ghee is clarified butter, which is extremely concentrated and a very powerful healing agent. It is normally used in the making up of herbal medicines, because it is made of pure creamy milk butter. It is also used in making beauty creams, potions, lotions, and other skin ointments.

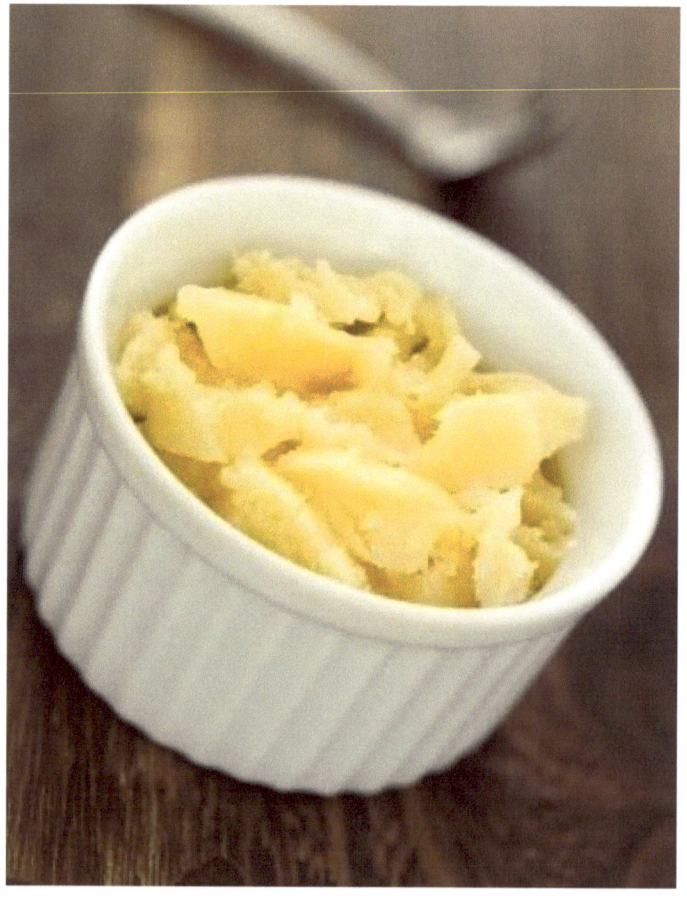

It has a powerful aroma, and that is why only just a spoonful is added to fry meats. It is going to float on the surface of the meat dish, after it has been cooked, so you need to stir the gravy before serving. Also, the food is not going to taste greasy, even though it looks like it has been swimming in fat.

Desi ghee is the concentrated form of pure butter, which is heated to reduce the butter of all the impurities as well as moisture. This concentrated butter is normally used in Eastern cuisine, for searing meat, sautéing, and frying food, because it offers a higher burning point.

You make this at home by taking 2 pounds of the best unsalted butter and melting it in a heavy bottomed pan. Allow the butter to liquefy on low heat for about 40 minutes. Maintain this simmering point, until all of the moisture in the butter has evaporated. The impurities are going to sink to the bottom of the pan. Remember to keep stirring the butter, so that it does not burn.

Pour off the clear butter and strain it through several thicknesses of muslin cloth. This butter is going to last for about a year, if it is placed in a cool and dry place. This butter is exorbitantly expensive. So in the East, people with easy access to plenty fresh milk make it right in their kitchens for crisp delicious frying results, and adding that taste of pure butter to all their dishes.

Conclusion

This book gives you plenty of information on how you can cure a number of ailments, naturally with milk and yogurt. For all those people who still have not managed to make yogurt a part of their daily diet, remember, yogurt is good for your gut.

Those drinks, which you buy from the market, supposedly full of probiotic bacteria is nothing but ordinary honest-to-goodness yogurt in expensive packages. This probiotic bacteria keeps your digestive system healthy and happy.

So cure yourself with milk and yogurt, Live Long and Prosper!

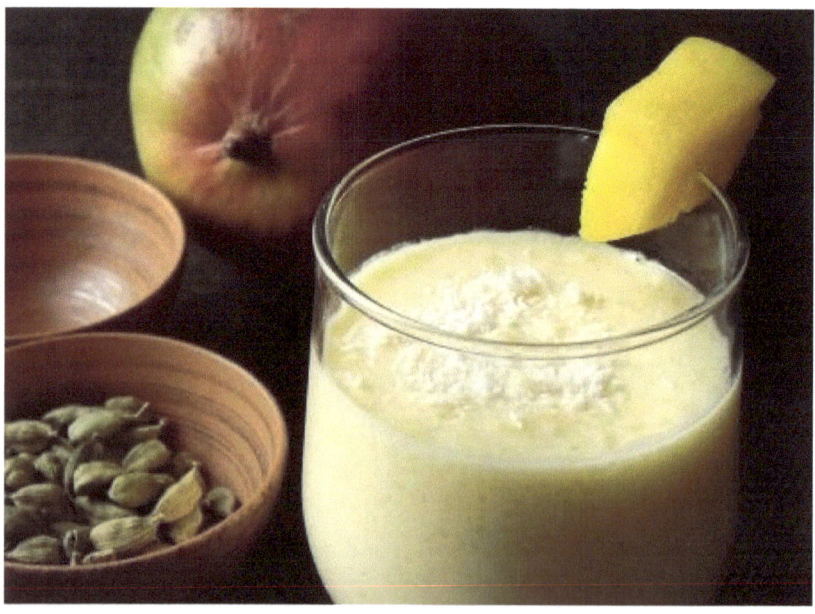

Author Bio

Dueep Jyot Singh is a Management and IT Professional who managed to gather Postgraduate qualifications in Management and English and Degrees in Science, French and Education while pursuing different enjoyable career options like being an hospital administrator, IT,SEO and HRD Database Manager/ trainer, movie , radio and TV scriptwriter, theatre artiste and public speaker, lecturer in French, Marketing and Advertising, ex-Editor of Hearts On Fire (now known as Solstice) Books Missouri USA, advice columnist and cartoonist, publisher and Aviation School trainer, ex-moderator on Medico.in, banker, student councilor ,travelogue writer … among other things!

One fine morning, she decided that she had enough of killing herself by Degrees and went back to her first love -- writing. It's more enjoyable! She already has 48 published academic and 14 fiction- in- different- genre books under her belt.

When she is not designing websites or making Graphic design illustrations for clients , she is browsing through old bookshops hunting for treasures, of which she has an enviable collection – including R.L. Stevenson, O.Henry, Dornford Yates, Maurice Walsh, De Maupassant, Victor Hugo, Sapper, C.N. Williamson, "Bartimeus" and the crown of her collection- Dickens "The Old Curiosity Shop," and "Martin Chuzzlewit" and so on… Just call her "Renaissance Woman" - collecting herbal remedies, acting like Universal Helping Hand/Agony Aunt, or escaping to her dear mountains for a bit of exploring, collecting herbs and plants, and trekking.

Check out some of the other JD-Biz Publishing books

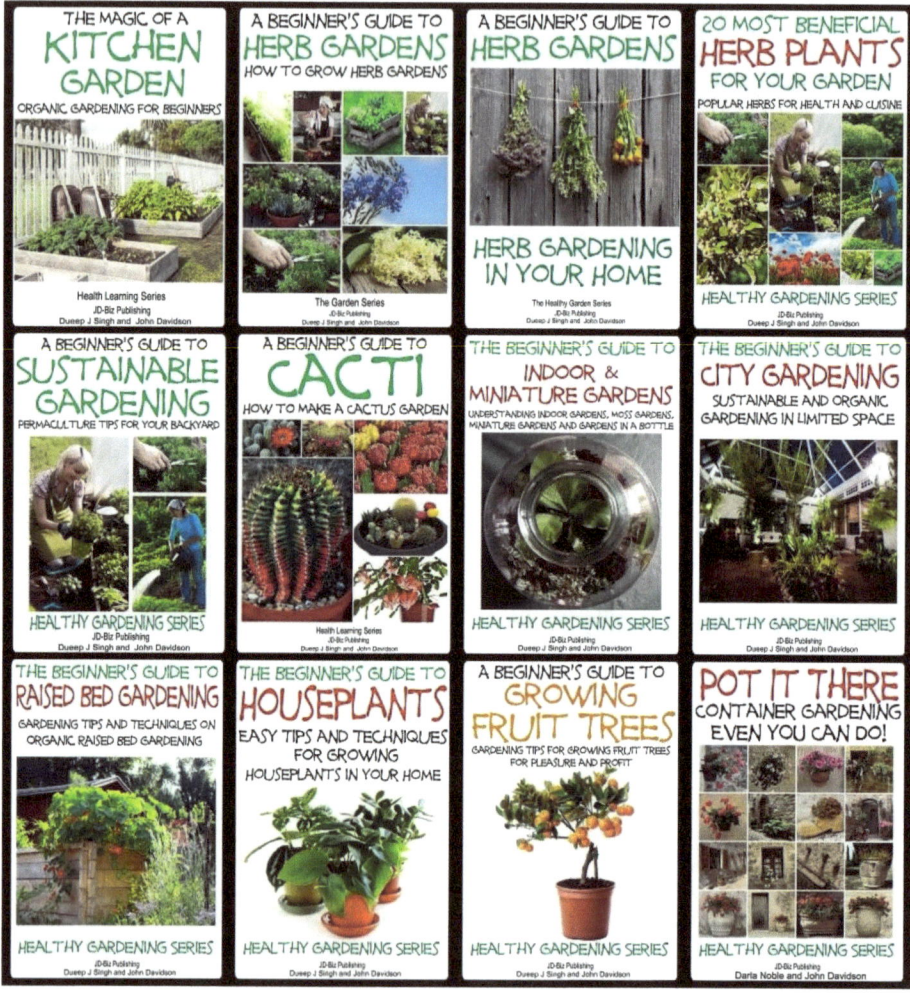

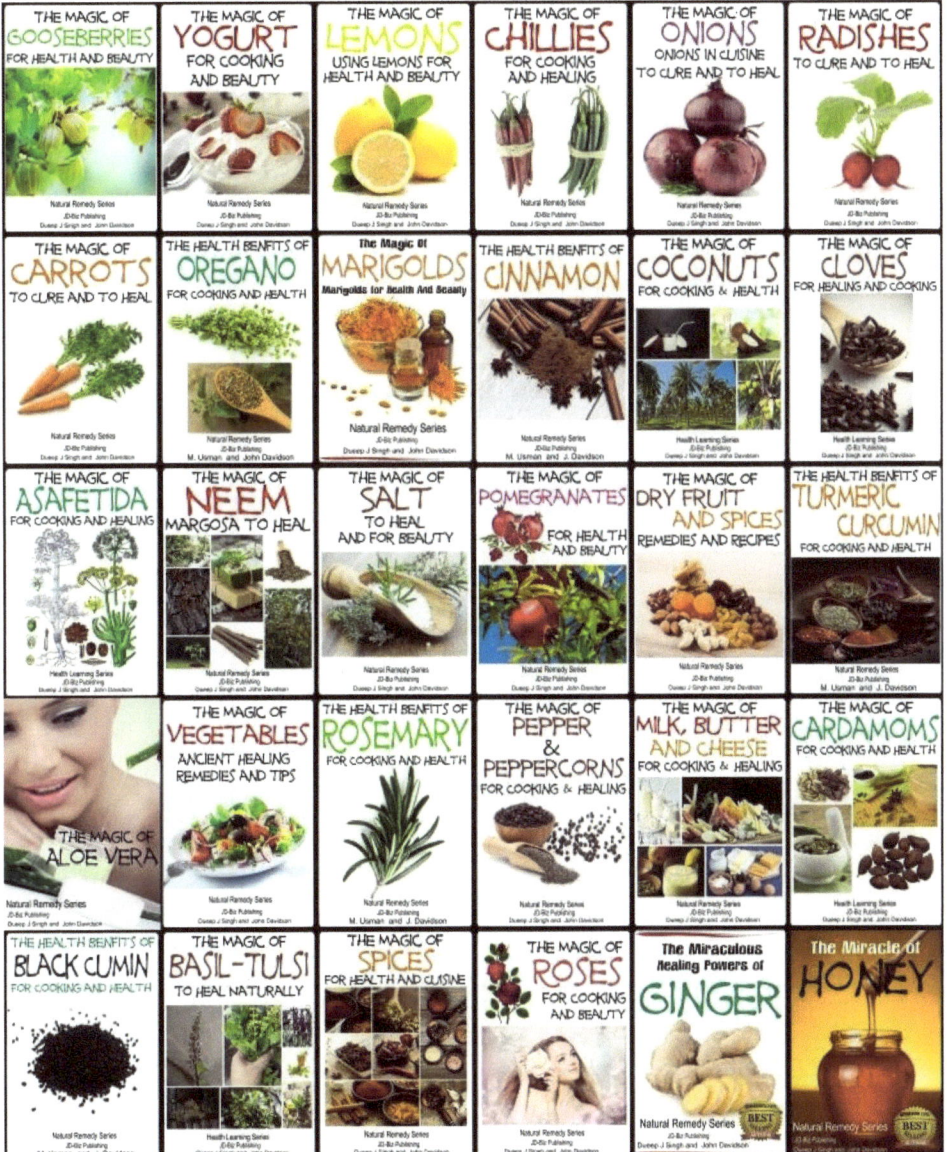

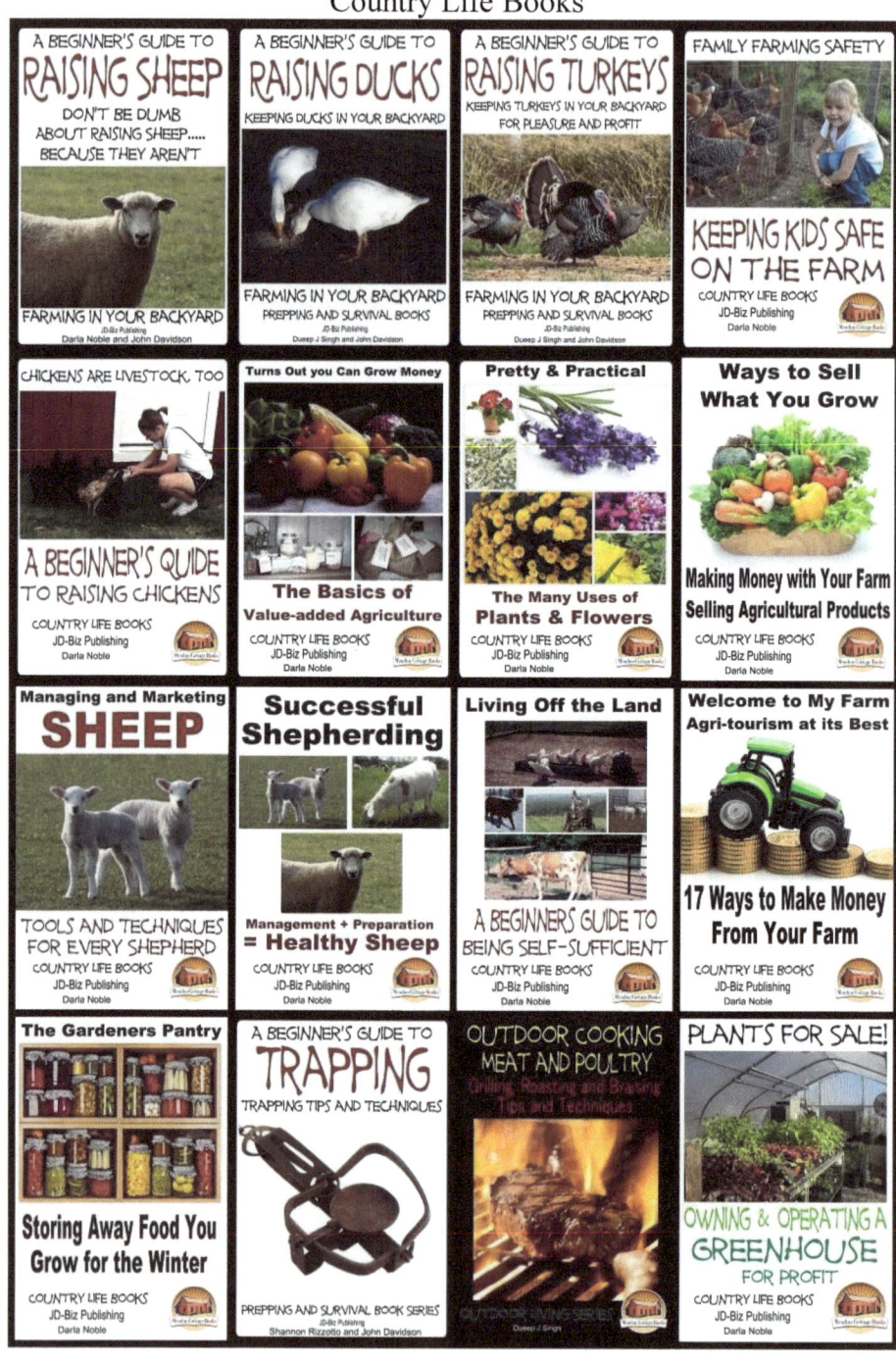

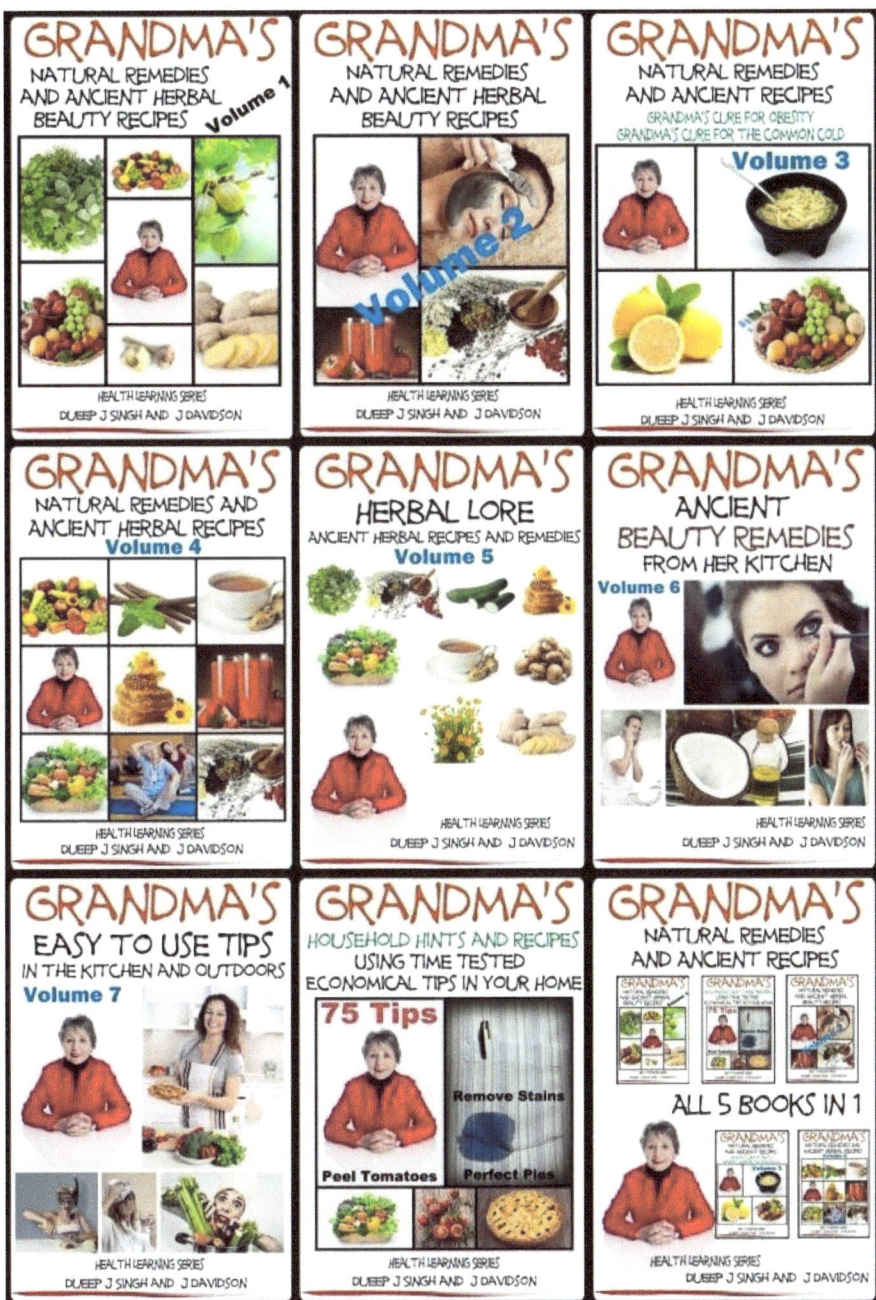

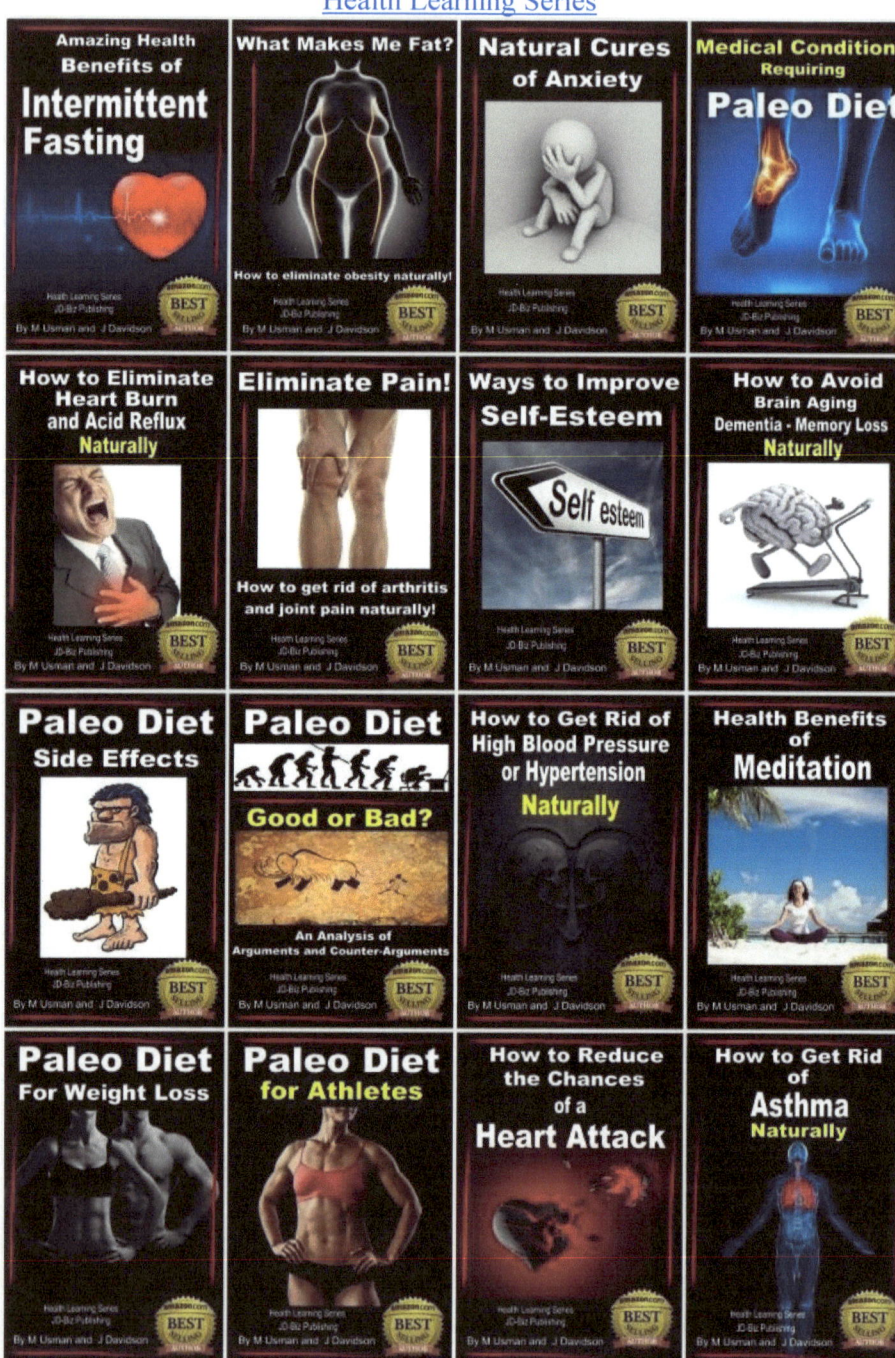

Amazing Animal Book Series

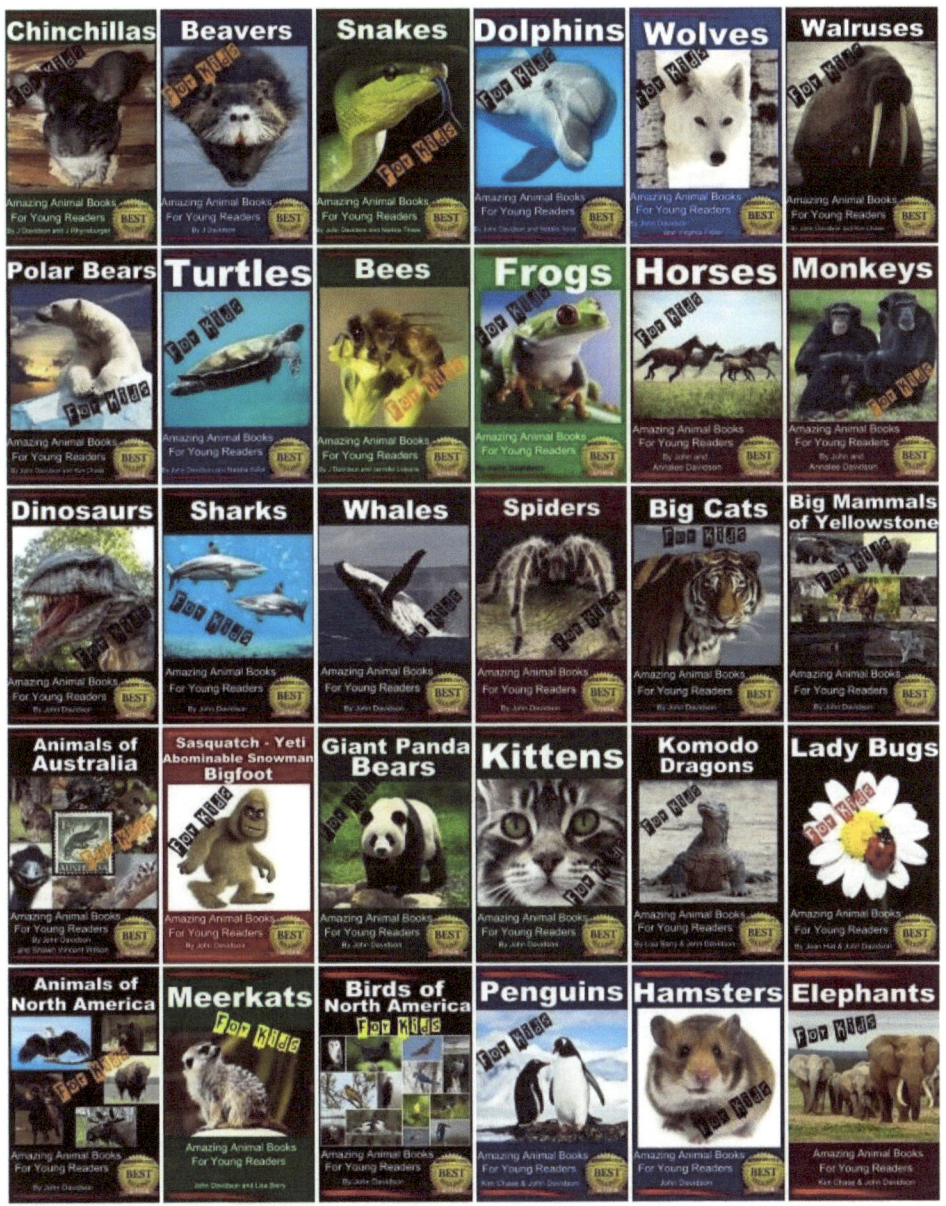

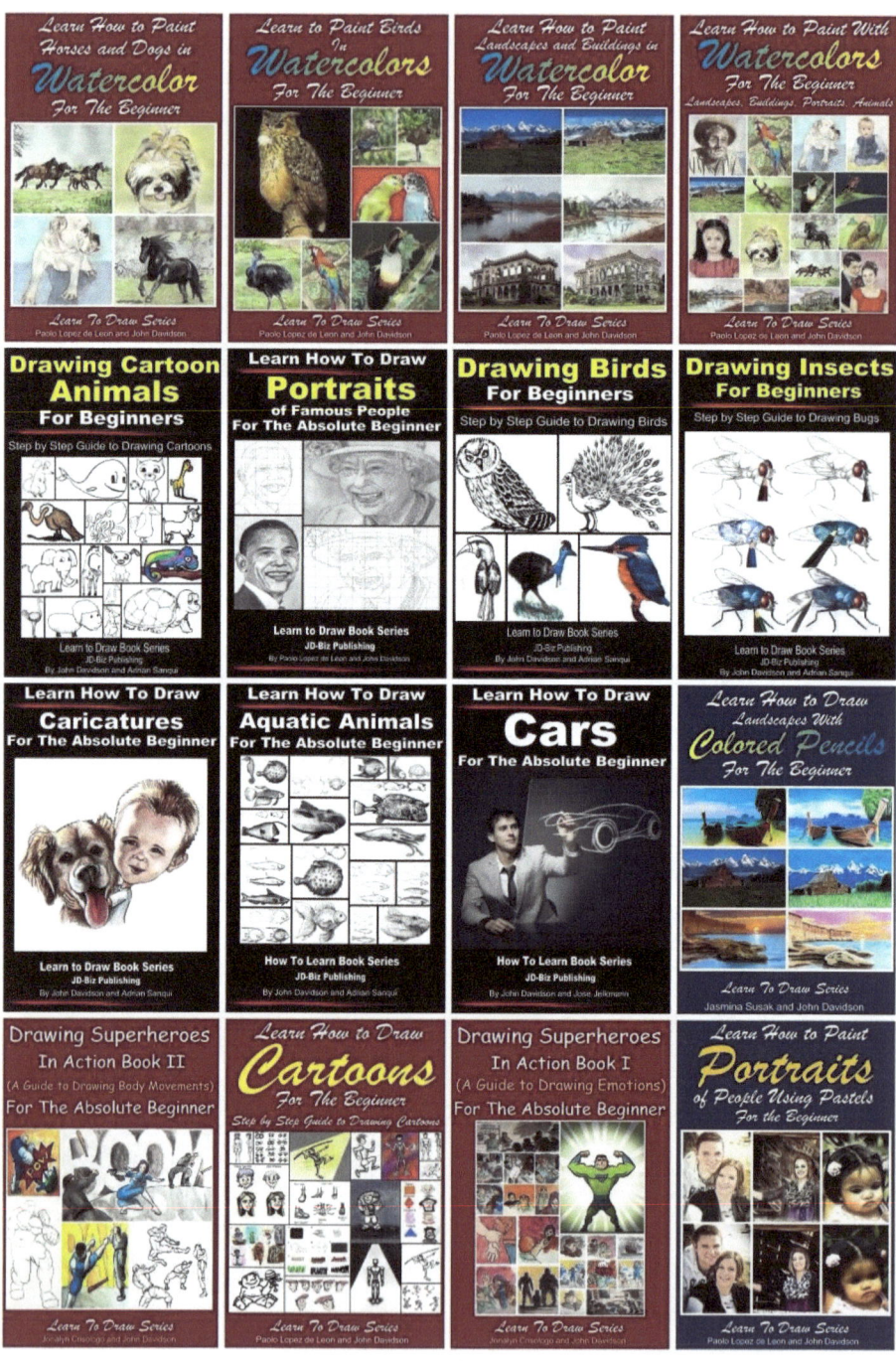

How to Build and Plan Books

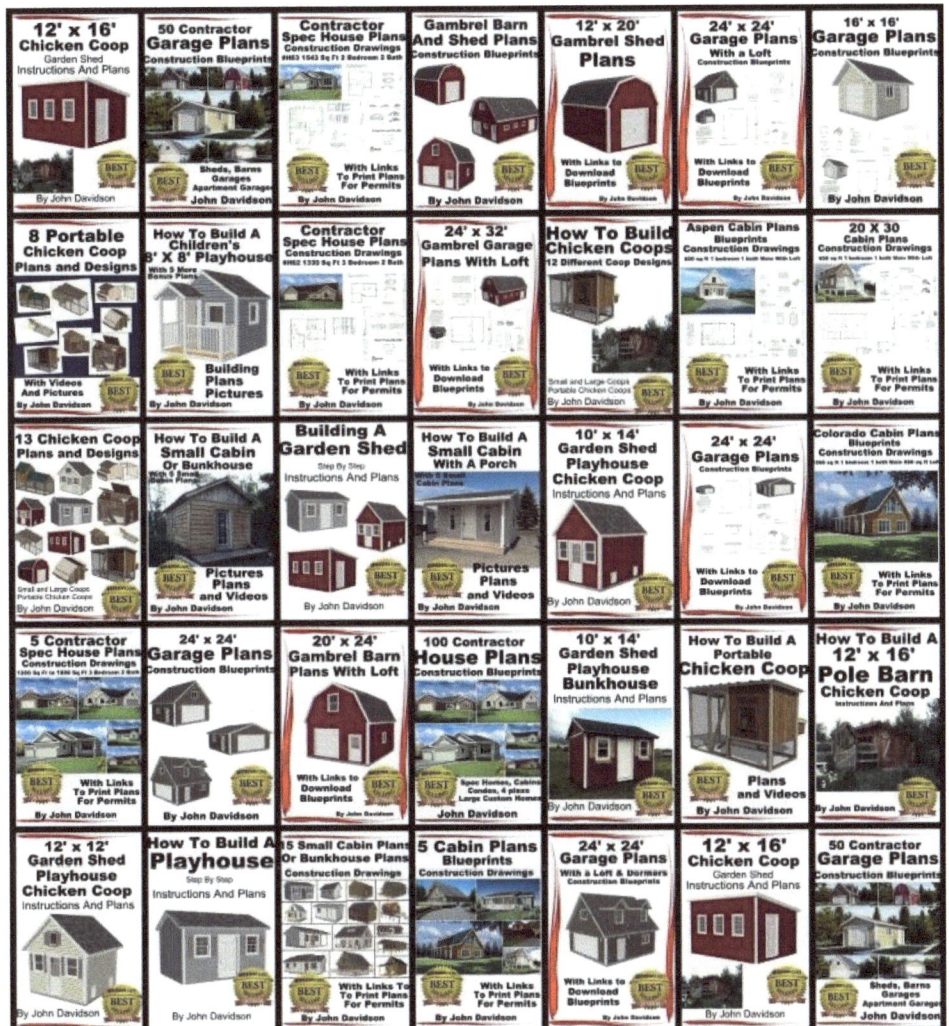

Entrepreneur Book Series

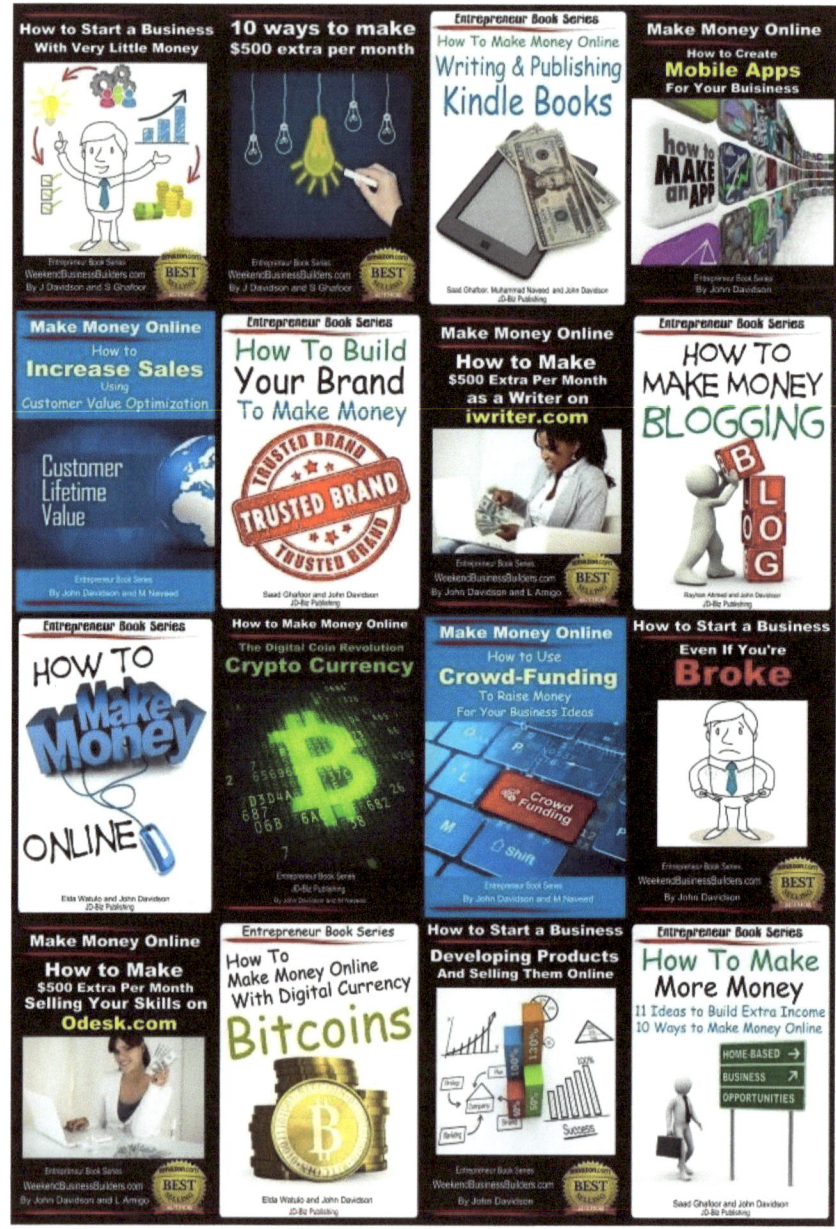

Our books are available at

1. Amazon.com

2. Barnes and Noble

3. Itunes

4. Kobo

5. Smashwords

6. Google Play Books

Download Free Books!

http://MendonCottageBooks.com

Publisher

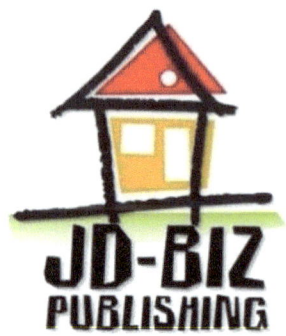

JD-Biz Corp

P O Box 374

Mendon, Utah 84325

http://www.jd-biz.com/

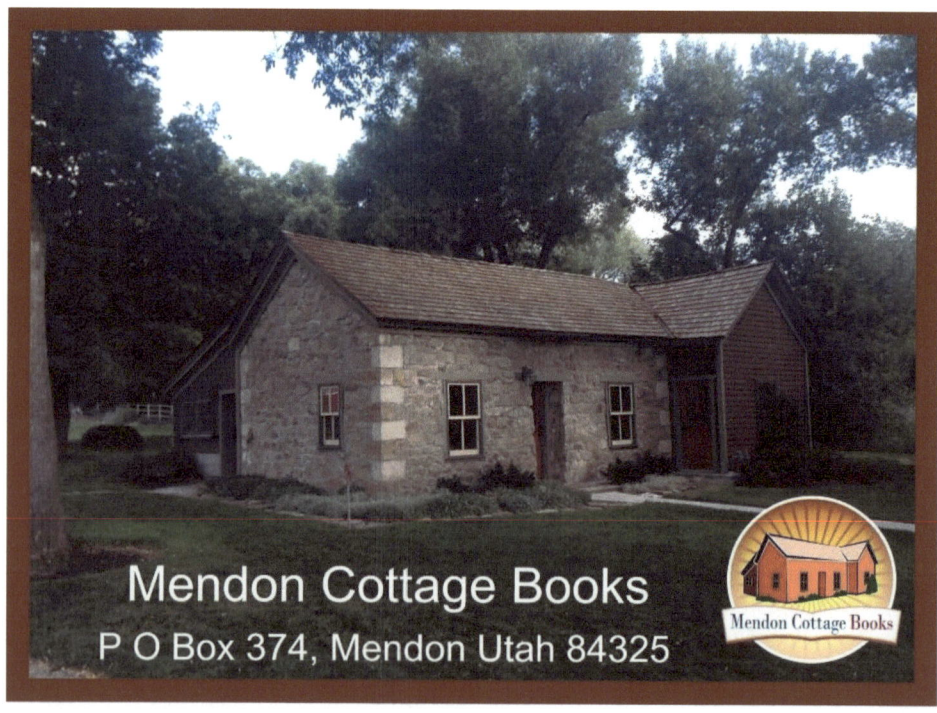